BIBLE CURE®

FOR

SKIN DISORDERS

DON COLBERT, M.D.

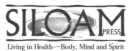

SILOAM PRESS

Living in Health—Body, Mind and Spirit

THE BIBLE CURE FOR SKIN DISORDERS
by Don Colbert, M.D.
Published by Siloam Press
A part of Strang Communications Company
600 Rinehart Road
Lake Mary, Florida 32746
www.siloampress.com

Unless otherwise noted, all Scripture quotations are from the Holy Bible, New Living Translation, copyright © 1996. Used by permission of Tyndale House Publishers, Inc., Wheaton, IL 60189. All rights reserved.

Scripture quotations marked KJV are from the King James Version of the Bible.

Scripture quotations marked NAS are from the New American Standard Bible. Copyright © 1960, 1962, 1963, 1968, 1971, 1972, 1973, 1975, 1977 by the Lockman Foundation. Used by permission. (www.Lockman.org)

Copyright © 2002 by Don Colbert, M.D.
All rights reserved

Library of Congress Catalog Card Number: 2002107794
International Standard Book Number: 0-88419-831-6

This book is not intended to provide medical advice or to take the place of medical advice and treatment from your personal physician. Readers are advised to consult their own doctors or other qualified health professionals regarding the treatment of their medical problems. Neither the publisher nor the author takes any responsibility for any possible consequences from any treatment, action or application of medicine, supplement, herb or preparation to any person reading or following the information in this book. If readers are taking prescription medications, they should consult with their physicians and not take themselves off of medicines to start supplementation without the proper supervision of a physician.

02 03 04 05 06 — 8 7 6 5 4 3 2 1
Printed in the United States of America

There's a Cleansing Fountain

The ancient Israelites experienced the pain of skin disorders. The prophet Isaiah described the affliction that God's people were experiencing: "You are sick from head to foot—covered with bruises, welts, and infected wounds—without any ointments or bandages" (Isa. 1:6).

God's people also experienced the power of God to heal and cleanse from disease and sin: "I have found a ransom; let his flesh become fresher than in youth, let him return to the days of his youthful vigor; then he will pray to God, and He will accept him, that he may see His face with joy, and He may restore His righteousness to man" (Job 33:24–26, NAS).

If you are experiencing skin disorders, you have not picked up this booklet by accident. I believe that God wants to reveal powerful truth about your condition that may surprise you. In addition, God wants to reveal to you a cleansing fountain that can heal the pain and discomfort of skin disorders. So get ready to explore some exciting truths.

Skin disorders affect nearly all of us sometime during our lives. They include various forms of acne, psoriasis and eczema. Approximately six mil-

> *"For I will restore you to health and I will heal you of your wounds," declares the LORD.*
> —JEREMIAH 30:17, NAS

lion people in the U.S. suffer from psoriasis, and about 2 percent of the world's population have psoriasis. Acne affects about 85 percent of all teenagers, and about one-fourth of them will have it so severely that they will be permanently scarred.[1]

Nevertheless, I have very good news for you. God wants you well, and He has provided wisdom and healing power to restore you.

Psoriasis, Eczema and Acne

This Bible Cure booklet discusses the cure for psoriasis, eczema and acne. You will discover that these three skin disorders have very similar root causes, effects and treatments. If you are suffering from one of these diseases, it will quickly become apparent to you that understanding all three will be of benefit.

This booklet is designed to bring healing to these skin disorders by first providing wisdom and understanding about the disorders themselves. Afterward, you will begin to understand that the natural, God-given cure involves strengthening you first through nutrition and supplements and through lifestyle changes, and then by strengthening your inner man through faith.

An Exciting First Step

No matter what the causes of your skin disorders, by picking up this Bible Cure booklet you have taken an exciting first step toward renewed health. God revealed His divine will for you through the apostle John, who wrote, "Beloved, I wish above all things that thou mayest prosper and be in health, even as thy soul prospereth" (3 John 2, kjv).

With God's help, you can begin walking in physical and spiritual renewal. So as you begin to read through the pages of this Bible Cure booklet, get ready to win! It is filled with hope and encouragement for understanding how to keep your body fit and healthy. In this book, you will

uncover God's divine plan of health
for body, soul and spirit,
through modern medicine, good nutrition,
and the medicinal power of
Scripture and prayer.

You will find key scripture passages throughout this book that will help you focus on the power of God. These divine promises will empower your prayers and redirect your thoughts to line up with God's plan of divine health for you—a plan that includes victory over skin disorders and their destructive physical and spiritual roots.

This Bible Cure booklet will give you a strategic plan for divine health in the following chapters:

If you are suffering with skin disorders, the chances are good that your body has been in a battle. Perhaps your mind and spirit have been, too.

With fresh confidence in the dynamic knowledge that God is real, that He is alive and that He loves you more than you could ever imagine, you can enjoy complete restoration of your health—body, mind and spirit.

It is my prayer that these powerful godly insights will bring health, wholeness and spiritual refreshing to you—body, mind and spirit. May they deepen your fellowship with God and strengthen your ability to worship and serve Him.

—Don Colbert, M.D.

Chapter 1

Clothed With Wisdom

God's wonderful wisdom is like a shield that covers and protects you—body, mind and spirit—from the daily assaults you encounter living in a hostile world. The Bible says, "Pay attention, my child, to what I say. Listen carefully. Don't lose sight of my words. Let them penetrate deep within your heart, for they bring life and radiant health to anyone who discovers their meaning" (Prov. 4:20–22).

If you are battling skin disorders, I have good news for you. God cares about everything that concerns you—nothing is too great or too small for God to heal. As a matter of fact, the Bible says that God's thoughts toward you are so numerous that you could never count them all, even if you tried. The psalmist wrote, "How precious are your thoughts about me, O God! They are innumerable!

I can't even count them; they outnumber the grains of sand!" (Ps. 139:17–18). His love for you is absolutely incomprehensible.

So, don't ever feel that God is too busy to be concerned about anything that afflicts you—body, mind or spirit. He loves you more than you could ever know.

Understanding Your Skin

As we discuss a few facts regarding psoriasis, acne and eczema, the understanding you gain will help you to make wise choices to put you on a path to healing and health. There are general principles that promote internal health, which is reflected in the health of your skin. And there are specific needs and treatments for each of these disorders that, when applied carefully, can result in healthy skin.

Since your first sunburn as a child, you have been aware that your skin is in layers, and that even though layers peeled off, there was "new" skin underneath. The marvel of our skin is one of the wonders that our Creator formed to endure for the entire length of our lives. It is constantly renewing itself to form the protective covering that it is for the rest of the body. However, when disease strikes the skin, it can cause great misery.

Your skin is the largest organ of the body, and it is made up of two main divisions: the epidermis and the dermis.

The epidermis

The epidermis is the thin outer layer of skin. It contains several layers of cells that gradually move up to the surface of the epidermis and become the protective layer of cells for our bodies. By the time these cells work their way up to your skin's surface, they have died. Your body eventually sheds these dead cells, similar to a snake shedding its skin. It takes about a month for the new layers of cells to move up through the epidermis and eventually be shed. In this way your amazing skin is able to regenerate each month.

The dermis

The second part of the skin, the dermis, is under the epidermis. It is made of elastic fibers and collagen, which give the skin tone and elasticity. This layer also contains fat, blood vessels, sweat glands, hair follicles and nerves. The dermis is thick and tougher than your epidermis layer, and it provides strength, tone and elasticity to your skin.

Skin disorders attack this amazing organ in a variety of ways, causing painful symptoms for those who suffer them.

Painful Psoriasis

Psoriasis is a chronic inflammatory skin disorder that results when skin cells reproduce too rapidly—at a rate approximately 1000 times greater than normal skin. Instead of normal regeneration that takes about a month, psoriasis skin cells regenerate every three or four days. In skin affected with psoriasis, both the epidermis and the dermis are affected by this abnormal cell division.[1]

The epidermis reacts to this abnormal cell reproduction by producing red patches covered with thick, silvery scales. These psoriatic lesions result simply from too many cells developing all at once. They often appear on the backs of the elbows and knees as well as on the scalp, lower back, buttocks, wrists and ankles.

Changes also occur in the dermis layer of skin as blood vessels become enlarged and engorged with blood.

> *And his flesh was restored like the flesh of a little child, and he was clean.*
> —2 KINGS 5:14, NAS

That is what makes the reddish color of patches

and plaques (raised patches) and causes them to bleed easily, especially when irritated.

When these patchy, scaly lesions appear, the skin has an increasingly difficult time performing its role as the protective barrier for your body. Body fluids are able to escape through the skin faster than they should, which can cause dehydration if enough surface area is involved. Certain nutritional deficiencies can also occur as a result.

Likely victims

Psoriasis is not gender biased—men and women develop this skin disorder almost equally. It does afflict Caucasians more readily, however, and is fairly uncommon in African Americans. The tendency to develop this disorder can be hereditary; if your parent has it, your risk of getting it is 25 percent. If both of your parents have psoriasis, your chance of getting it increases to 50 percent. Generally, this skin disorder first starts to show up between the ages of fifteen and thirty-five.

Types of psoriasis

There are several types of psoriasis, and symptoms vary with each type. The most common is the *plaque-type psoriasis,* which is marked by red, raised lesions with clear borders and silvery scales. This is the type that typically breaks out on the knees, elbows, scalp and lower back. *Guttate psoriasis* appears as red droplets, usually on the arms, legs or trunk. *Flexural* or *inverse psoriasis* usually develops in skin folds such as the armpits, the crease of the buttocks, under the breasts or in the groin area. These lesions usually appear red and inflamed, but generally don't scale.

Erythrodermic psoriasis usually affects the entire body, covering it with a red, scaly, highly itchy rash. And *pustular psoriasis* happens when psoriatic blisters appear on the skin. These blisters are filled with white blood cells commonly known as "pus." The lesions are not infected, and they are not contagious.

About 10 percent of patients who suffer with psoriasis develop a type of arthritis called *psoriatic arthritis.* It usually affects the fingers, but it can involve other joints, too.

Cause of psoriasis

No one knows the exact cause of psoriasis, although many researchers now believe that psoriasis is a type of autoimmune disease, which is a disease that causes a person's body to begin attacking itself. Psoriasis is a type of autoimmune disorder that is *T-cell mediated.* T-cells are white blood cells that are supposed to protect us by helping our bodies mount an immune response. In patients with psoriasis, T-cells multiply rapidly and trigger skin cells to begin regenerating at an accelerated pace, similar to wound healing. Normally when T-cells finish their job, they stop multiplying. However, this does not occur in psoriasis; hence, the skin disorder occurs, though the cause is not clear.

Proper cell division is dependent, in part, on a balance between cyclic AMP and cyclic GMP (two internal controllers in the cell). Cyclic AMP regulates the metabolism, keeping it from regenerating too fast. An excess

> O LORD my God, you have done many miracles for us. Your plans for us are too numerous to list. If I tried to recite all your wonderful deeds, I would never come to the end of them.
> —PSALM 40:5

of cyclic GMP in a cell causes it to regenerate too fast. It is important to balance these two "comptrollers." In order to control psoriasis, scientists wanted to discover what prevents the body from producing enough cyclic AMP and what causes it to produce too much cyclic GMP. Some answers are forthcoming.

Triggering an outbreak

Many factors seem to have the power to trigger an outbreak of psoriasis or to aggravate an outbreak that has begun. Psoriatic skin is much more prone to a breakout if it's exposed to trauma, irritation or prolonged pressure or friction. For example, a skin injury or trauma, ranging from an insect sting or bite to a burn or cut, can aggravate psoriasis. Even prolonged pressure from sitting, kneeling or leaning on your elbow for a prolonged period of time can trigger the outbreak.

Emotional stress can cause an outbreak of psoriasis. Infections such as strep throat, as well as medications (including steroids, anti-inflammatory medications like Advil or Aleve, beta-blockers and antimalarials), may also trigger psoriasis. And certain foods, such as nightshade vegetables (tomatoes, peppers, potatoes and eggplant), can trigger an outbreak of psoriasis. Fried foods, hydrogenated fats, red meats, pork and alcohol are all common triggers for psoriasis.

Science has also discovered that incomplete digestion of protein can trigger an attack of psoriasis and can aggravate an already existing outbreak. When your body is not able to digest proteins completely, excessive amounts of polypeptides, amino acids and other products of protein digestion begin to accumulate in the small intestines. The bacteria that live there metabolize these protein compounds into toxic substances called *polyamines*. Psoriasis sufferers usually have elevated levels of these toxic substances.

These polyamines keep your body from making enough cyclic AMP to control normal

> *My bone clings to my skin and my flesh.*
> —JOB 19:20, NAS

cell regeneration. Without this important regulator of metabolism, certain skin cells (like those at the elbows and knees) begin proliferating up to a thousand times faster than normal cell division.

All of these triggers emphasize our need to understand the wisdom God has provided to keep the delicate balance of our skin regulators functioning for health.

Addressing Issues of Acne

Acne is one skin disorder that has made young people miserable for many generations. How many young girls have purchased a prom dress and everything required for a perfect evening, only to wake up in the morning to an outbreak of acne? How many young boys have suffered the teasing and unkind remarks of peers who do not suffer from acne?

Drug treatments that offer relief from symptoms of acne can have harmful side effects that you may choose to avoid. If you suffer from any form of acne, it may relieve you to learn that even the worst cases of acne can be treated by natural methods with very good results.

A difficult disease

Acne, the most common of all skin disorders, is actually an inflammatory disease of the sebaceous glands and hair follicles of the skin, resulting from dead, sticky skin cells that are retained inside the skin's pores and that form impactions. The entire surface of your skin, except for your palms and the soles of your feet, is covered with small skin pores (also called follicles). Each pore is actually a tiny opening to a small tube that runs through the skin's epidermis layer into the dermis. This hair follicle contains a hair as well as sebaceous glands that manufacture a type of oil called sebum.

The hair may be so small that it's actually invisible to the naked eye, while other pores grow a thicker type of hair and are responsible for areas of our body that are covered with hair. The visible or invisible hair acts as a wick to expel oil, dead cells and other debris out of the pores. As long as these pores function efficiently, they help to maintain healthy skin throughout your lifetime. However, during puberty, the production of oil (sebum) greatly increases with hormone production, specifically testosterone, in both boys and girls. Testosterone triggers the follicles usually on the face, chest, back and shoulders to enlarge and to produce more oil or sebum, which can sometimes create problems.

Cause of acne

The follicle of an acne patient is actually producing cells at an accelerated rate, approximately five times faster than normal. When the cells die, they collect inside the pores, forming impactions. These cells, along with their oily sebaceous secretions, then begin to stick together and form an impaction inside the pore. As more dead skin cells inside the pore are being sloughed off, the impaction grows larger and larger. Bacteria are present in all follicles. However, as more oil accumulates in this impacted pore, more bacteria begin to multiply.

Though we know how acne impactions are formed, the cause of acne is unknown. However, predisposing factors include hereditary tendencies as well as the hormonal imbalance of puberty we have mentioned. Specific inciting factors may include food allergies, endocrine disorders, therapy with adrenal corticosteroid hormones and psychogenic factors.

Vitamin deficiencies, ingestion of halogens and contact with chemicals such as tar and chlorinated hydrocarbons may be specific causative factors. The fact that bacteria are important once the disease is present is indicated by the successful results following antibiotic therapy.[2]

Likely victims

Many of us believe that acne is only the scourge of teens, but it can persist in about 30 percent of people in adult life. Sadly, 5 percent of women and 1 percent of men are still battling acne at age forty.[3]

Acne rosacea, a chronic eruption usually on the cheeks and nose, is seen almost exclusively in adults over thirty years of age; it affects women three times as often as men. Most individuals with rosacea have a dramatic flushing reaction, especially in response to alcohol, spicy foods, hot drinks, sunlight, hot flashes from menopause and emotional stimuli.

Enduring Eczema

Eczema (also called dermatitis) is an inflammation of the skin that usually results in scaling, flaking, thickening, color changes and sometimes itching. There are various types of eczema:

- *Atopic dermatitis* is a hereditary form that sometimes becomes apparent in infancy but may occur initially late in life. It usually appears on the face, in the bends of the elbows and behind the knees and is marked by itching.

- *Seborrhea* is a form of dermatitis characterized by greasy scales occurring on the scalp as dandruff and sometimes affecting the eyebrows, nasolabial folds and eyelids.

- *Nummular eczema* forms coinlike lesions, most commonly located on the arms, back, buttocks and lower legs.

- *Dyshidrotic eczema* is characterized by irritation of the skin of the palms of the hands and soles of the feet. It occurs especially between the fingers and is associated with blisters that burn and itch.

- *Contact dermatitis* is an inflammatory condition of the skin caused from irritants such as detergents, acids and solvents. Another form of contact dermatitis is allergic contact dermatitis, which is commonly caused by poison ivy, poison oak, poison sumac and nickel, which is often present in cheap jewelry.

While we cannot list all the forms of eczema, the treatment for the most common form, atopic dermatitis, will also help to relieve the other forms of eczema.

Cause of eczema (dermatitis)

No class, age or sex is exempt, but persons with thin, dry skin are more susceptible. Again, there is not a known cause for the various forms of eczema. There may be allergic, hereditary or psychological components. It is clear that symptoms are made worse by contact with wool, climactic changes and excessive exposure to soap, water and oils.

Nummular eczema is often associated with dry skin and worsens in dry weather. And the cause for dyshidrotic eczema may be associated with contact allergy or a fungal infection.

Good News: Treatable and Beatable

By now you realize that there are many skin disorders that any one individual may have. The good news is that even if you have suffered with a skin disorder for many years, and even if your problem is very severe, it is both treatable and beatable. Wise nutritional and lifestyle choices made in response to suggestions given here can begin to turn your situation around.

Some minor natural lifestyle changes, including diet, nutritional supplements and a fresh, clear vision of God's boundless love and care for you, can make all the difference in the world. For some, it can provide a brand-new start.

So, if you have a skin disorder, even a very serious one, be encouraged. In the next several chapters we will discuss how applying God's won-

> *When evildoers came upon me to devour my flesh, my adversaries and my enemies, they stumbled and fell.*
> —PSALM 27:2, NAS

derful wisdom, a dash of faith in His limitless love and the power of His Word can leave you feeling and looking brand-new. God's wisdom will refresh your body and clothe your skin with vibrant health, so others will say of you, "His [or her] flesh was restored like the flesh of a little child" (2 Kings 5:14, NAS).

A BIBLE CURE PRAYER
FOR YOU

Dear Lord, thank You for restoring and refreshing me—body, soul and spirit. I thank You that Your cleansing and refreshing power extends to the largest organ on my body—my skin. In Your wonderful Word, You promise to heal all of my diseases. Therefore, I give You my skin disorder and ask You for cleansing, healing and restoration. I thank You that there's nothing about me that's too great or too small for Your tender care and loving concern. I receive Your healing power right now. Open my heart and mind, and plant Your wisdom into my soul so that I will walk in a brand-new path of health. Amen.

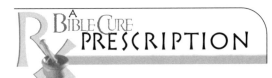

A BIBLE CURE PRESCRIPTION

Describe your skin disorder.

_____

_____

_____

_____

According to the various categories provided in this chapter, which skin disorder, or disorders, do you believe you have?

_____

_____

_____

_____

Chapter 2

Glowing Through Nutrition

We live in a time in which many of the laws that God instituted to protect our health have been completely ignored. These include laws for farming recorded in the Old Testament to make certain that our food would supply an abundance of nutrition to our bodies.

God warned us that if we ignored His healthy principles for living, our health could suffer. He even mentioned diseases (which sound a lot like the skin disorders we are discussing—boils of Egypt, tumors, scurvy and the itch) that would be a result of disobedience to His laws (Deut. 28:27). Our wise and wonderful Creator tried to teach us many, many years ago that the way we nourish our bodies is a major key to health.

God loves you so much that He doesn't want you to suffer poor health. The Bible says, "For he doth not afflict willingly nor grieve the children of men" (Lam. 3:33, KJV). Yet, God also declared through His prophet, "My people are destroyed for lack of knowledge" (Hos. 4:6, KJV). As we seek His wisdom concerning our bodies, He will be faithful to fulfill His healing promises.

Nutritional Regimen

Our discussion of a healthy protocol for eating can bring healing to people suffering from a skin disorder of any type. There are some specifics for particular disorders that will be discussed separately, as well.

Toxic overload

You may know that your liver is a giant filter that purifies your body of toxins, poisons, environmental chemicals and anything else that could harm your body. One of the problems with living in today's world is that our livers must work much harder to cleanse our bodies from all of the toxins we encounter daily. When your liver starts to fall behind on its work, the body becomes toxic and subject to disease.

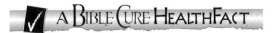

Your Valiant Liver

Your liver performs more than five hundred different functions. Every minute, about two quarts of blood is filtered through your liver. When this powerful organ is working efficiently, it filters out about 99 percent of the bacteria and other poisonous toxins from your blood. With poor eating habits as well as environmental pollution affecting our bodies, many times the liver cannot catch up on its internal housekeeping. In that case, the body cannot resist disease and will react with symptoms that reveal your particular weaknesses, such as skin disorders.

HEALTHFACT HEALTHFACT HEALTHFACT HEALTHFACT HEALTHFACT HEALTHFACT HEALTHFACT

That's why, if you are suffering a skin disorder, it is not only important for you to heal the intestinal tract, but also to begin providing adequate nutrition for your liver to help it catch up on its internal detoxification.

Digestion problems

Poor digestion also tends to aggravate disease, especially psoriasis. Usually with poor digestion comes increased "intestinal permeability." This is a term for microscopic holes appearing along the walls of your small intestine that allow food that hasn't been completely digested to pass right into your bloodstream. These toxins go directly into the liver, undermining your liver's role of detoxification and triggering the release of free radicals, which puts even more strain on your liver. This condition is sometimes called "leaky gut" because your gut actually leaks toxic substances into your bloodstream. It leads to food allergies, food sensitivities and autoimmune diseases. Not surprising, it is very common in those who have skin disorders.

Leaky gut can be a factor in yeast overgrowth inside the intestines. Yeast toxins lead to an increase in cyclic GMP levels within the

> *Now those who belong to Christ Jesus have crucified the flesh with its passions and desires.*
> —GALATIANS 5:24, NAS

skin, which in turn leads to an increased growth of skin cells. Candida overgrowth is common in many people with skin disorders. Most patients with skin disorders can benefit from the candida diet as well as by taking nystatin, which kills intestinal candida. (For more information, please refer to *The Bible Cure for Candida and Yeast Infections.*)

Food allergies

Leaky gut and candida can also create food allergies, food sensitivities and food triggers for skin disorders. Two-thirds of your immune system is actually located in your digestive or GI tract. When you develop leaky gut, candida or bacterial overgrowth, your immune system can begin to mistake a harmless substance, like food, for a dangerous foreign invader.

In response, it launches an all-out attack against this harmless molecule of food. That is what triggers most food allergies and sensitivities. Many of my patients with skin disorders also suffer from food allergies. For many, certain foods actually trigger psoriasis, even though they may not be allergic to that food.

Common food allergies

To begin a nutritional approach to treating your skin disorder, the following food groups that are the most common cause of food allergies, sensitivities and triggers for skin disorders should be eliminated for three months:

- Nightshades, such as tomatoes, peppers, potatoes and eggplant

- Dairy products, including yogurt

- Alcohol, including red wine, beer and spirits

- Hydrogenated fats, partially hydrogenated fats and fried foods

- Red meat and pork (especially bacon)

- Vinegar

- Gluten (found in all wheat products: breads, crackers, wheat cereals, bagels and pretzels), as well as oats, rye, barley, gravies, soups, etc.

- Sweets and processed foods like white flour, white rice, sugary cereals, etc.

Some psoriasis patients are also sensitive to eggs, corn, soy, chocolate, caffeine, peanuts, citrus, strawberries and food colorings and flavorings. After eliminating these foods for three months, along with following the nutritional protocol recommended in this book, many patients discover that their skin returns to normal.

After three months, you may begin to reintroduce one of these foods every four days. If your skin reacts, you will know for sure that you are still sensitive to that particular food and that it should be eliminated for good. To help you figure out to which foods you react, you can perform a rotational diet or have food allergy testing by a lab such as ImmunoLabs in Ft. Lauderdale, Florida. Your physician can order this test by calling (800) 231-9197. (For more information on food allergies, please refer to *The Bible Cure for Allergies.*)

Other considerations

If you are like most Americans, you probably eat way too much saturated fat. These fats are found in fatty cuts of meat, skins of chicken and turkey, dairy products, fried foods and processed meats (such as hot dogs, bacon, bologna, pepperoni and salami).

Other nutritional deficiencies commonly encountered in those with skin disorders include vitamins A and B deficiencies, as well as a lack of zinc and

> *Let his flesh become fresher than in youth, let him return to the days of his youthful vigor.*
> —JOB 33:25, NAS

selenium. And you may also be deficient in Omega-3 fatty acids (fish oils) and GLA.

Nutritional Regimen

This nutritional regimen will be helpful especially for psoriasis and eczema patients, as well as patients suffering from acne.

- Avoid food triggers and allergies as discussed above. An elimination diet that excludes these common offenders for three months and adds them back into your diet one by one is very effective to determine which foods trigger a reaction in you.

- If you have candida overgrowth, which is fairly common, follow the candida diet as outlined in *The Bible Cure for Candida and Yeast Infections.* If you score high on the yeast questionnaire found in that booklet, it is likely that you are suffering from candida and will need to avoid all moldy foods as well as all sugary foods.

- It's also important to decrease foods that are high in arachidonic acid, including red meat, pork, dairy products and egg yolks.

- If you do not have candida, I recommend that you follow a balanced eating plan, with 40 percent carbohydrates, 30 percent protein and 30 percent good fats, which is discussed in my book *Walking in Divine Health* (Siloam Press, 1999).

- For carbohydrates, make sure you chose whole grains, fresh vegetables and low-glycemic fruits such as Granny Smith apples, kiwi, grapefruits, blueberries, blackberries and raspberries. Some psoriasis patients are sensitive to grapefruit and strawberries.

- For proteins, choose from free-range chicken and turkey without skins, salmon, mackerel, herring, pompano and sardines two to three times a week. Avoid red meat and pork, especially bacon. I recommend protein supplements such as soy, whey or rice protein. Also, make sure that you take a digestive enzyme such as Divine Health Digestive Enzyme in order to help you adequately digest the protein.

- For fats, choose from cold-pressed vegetable oils found at health food stores, almonds (not slivered), macadamia nuts and most other seeds and nuts (except peanuts and cashews). Also good are avocados, olives, extra-virgin olive oil, flaxseeds (that you grind in a coffee grinder), flaxseed oil, evening primrose oil, borage oil, black currant oil and fish oil.

By eating a 40-30-30 diet, you will balance your nutritional intake so that it will dramatically decrease the amount of arachidonic acid that is formed by the body. Also, it will be necessary to avoid bad fats: fried foods, hydrogenated and partially hydrogenated fats, and polyunsaturated fats (heat processed) found in most vegetable oils purchased at the grocery store. These bad fats are triggers for skin disorders, especially psoriasis.

If you are faithful to this natural Bible cure and your skin disorder does not start to clear, you will need to have food allergy testing by ImmunoLabs.

Acidic overload

If the 40-30-30 diet, the candida diet and elimination of trigger foods does not bring improvement to your skin disorder, you may also need to bring your body into balance in respect to acidity. You will need to increase your consumption of alkaline foods. Many Americans, and most patients with psoriasis, have acid overload of the tissues.

Most Americans eat too many acid-producing foods such as processed foods, meats, sugary foods, fried foods and so forth. They also consume inadequate amounts of alkaline-producing foods such as fruits and vegetables. The result is that the tissues of the body tend to become more acidic rather than neutral or slightly alkaline as they need to be. This acidic condition makes it more difficult for nutrients to enter into the cells and for metabolic waste and toxins to be eliminated from the cells.

As we have mentioned, patients with skin disorders often have a liver that is already very toxic. Therefore, eating more alkaline foods will help cleanse the tissues of the body, which in turn may help relieve the skin condition.

A few simple ways to create a healthy alkaline balance include:

- Make it a point to eat at least 1 cup of greens (for example, kale, mustard, turnip, collard or endive) daily.

- Eat alkalizing grains like oats, quinoa and wild rice.

- Enjoy liberal amounts of fruits.

Specifics for psoriasis

Research has shown that many patients with psoriasis are lacking adequate amounts of GLA, an activated essential fatty acid, in their diets. Also, eating hydrogenated fats, suffering viral infections and experiencing too much stress diminish the supply of GLA. There are only a few sources of GLA, including oatmeal, evening primrose oil, borage oil and black currant oil.

Researchers have also found that psoriasis lesions contain much higher levels of free arachidonic acid, a fatty acid that may be largely to blame for much of your psoriasis troubles. To lower the levels of arachidonic acid, it is especially important to avoid all sugars and to decrease dramatically the amount of processed carbohydrates in your diet such as white bread, white rice, potatoes and corn. Also, avoid foods high in arachidonic acid, such as red meats, pork, dairy products and egg yolks. Following the 40-30-30 plan will be very healing to your condition as well.

Unfortunately, itching is one of the very unpleasant side effects of psoriasis and eczema that can continue day and night. You will need to keep your skin well hydrated by drinking plenty of water. These skin disorders may actually dehydrate the skin very quickly. To make sure you are drinking enough water, divide your body weight in pounds by two. Drink that amount of ounces a day of filtered water. For example, if you weigh 100 pounds, which divided by two equals 50, you would drink 50 ounces of water a day. Keeping your body hydrated properly will relieve many other disease symptoms as well.

A word of caution: It's commonly known that drinking alcohol will make your psoriasis worse. Alcohol places an even greater strain on your already overwhelmed liver, and it can damage the lining of the GI tract.

Specifics for eczema

Studies show that breast-feeding infants protects them against atopic dermatitis (the most common form of eczema), especially if the baby is breast-fed for the first few months of life. In addition, infants who are breast-fed and do develop atopic dermatitis generally suffer a much less severe case. This fact could be helpful for parents who have eczema and desire to protect their children from it.

The most common food allergens triggering atopic dermatitis are dairy products, eggs and peanuts. These three foods accounted for approximately 80 percent of all cases of the disorder in children.[1]

Other problem foods associated with atopic dermatitis include tomatoes, wheat, soybeans, corn, chicken, food colorings (especially yellow), preservatives (especially benzoate), fish, citrus and chocolate.

Specifics for acne

Foods high in iodine as well as vitamin supplements containing a lot of iodine can aggravate acne. Since iodine is added to table salt, over-salting your food can contribute to the disease. For that reason, packaged chips, pizzas and most fast foods should be avoided.

Foods that contain hormones, such as milk, butter, cheese, ice cream and fatty cuts of meat such as beef and pork, may also

> *Who pardons all your iniquities; who heals all your diseases.*
> —PSALM 103:3, NAS

cause acne to flare. There's a myth that says acne is caused by fatty foods, fried foods and chocolate. However, studies have not confirmed that myth.

Eating a balanced diet and avoiding the foods outlined above will have a cleansing effect on the system and, along with drinking plenty of fresh water, will bring welcome relief for acne sufferers.

If you have acne rosacea, it's important for you to avoid foods that will make your blood vessels dilate, or vasodilating foods. These include alcohol, spicy foods—especially salsas—coffee, hot tea and other hot beverages and any other foods that cause you to flush. You may need to keep a food diary to determine the foods that cause flushing. In addition, I also commonly place my patients with acne rosacea on a candida diet, as mentioned above.

Receiving divine help

What you eat really matters—especially when you have a skin disorder that's directly linked to your diet. God will help you to make the changes in your eating habits that you need to make to be healed. The Bible says that when people cry to Him in their trouble, "he saveth them out of their distresses. He sent his word, and healed them, and delivered them from their destructions" (Ps. 107:19–20, κjv).

If you will place your eating habits on the altar of God and surrender to Him all your choices regarding foods, you will receive His divine help to overcome any damaging eating habits you may have developed over the years.

There's no disease that He cannot or will not heal. Psalm 103:3 declares, "He forgives all my sins and heals all my diseases." That's great news!

A BIBLE CURE PRAYER
FOR YOU

Dear Lord, I thank You that You are the Lord of healing—of the body, soul and spirit. Help me to be faithful to sound wisdom about my diet. I place all of my bad dietary habits on Your altar, and I give my will to You in matters having to do with what I choose to eat. Empower me to eat in a way that is consistent with my own good health. In Jesus' name, amen.

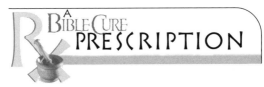

R A BIBLE CURE PRESCRIPTION

Create a diet for yourself for the next month based upon the above information for your particular skin disorder. Use a calendar on which you can write the foods you want to eat each week. Make it enjoyable, and reward yourself for fulfilling each day of the special healing diet. List below several healthy rewards you will give yourself.

_____

_____

_____

_____

_____

Write a prayer asking for wisdom to help you plan the diet and strength to complete it.

_____

_____

_____

Chapter 3

Beautifying With Supplements

G od expects you to nourish your body and to treat it with love and respect. The Bible says, "No one hates his own body but lovingly cares for it, just as Christ cares for his body, which is the church" (Eph. 5:29). One of the important ways to care for your body is to be sure that it is receiving all of the nutrients that it requires for health.

Supplements are a powerful way to be sure that your body's largest organ, your skin, is getting all that it needs to battle skin disorders. In addition, supplement power can help support healing and restore the beauty of normal skin function.

Soothing Supplements for Psoriasis and Eczema

As you begin your supplement program, it will be very helpful to test for polyamines, those toxic compounds formed in the GI tract as a result of incomplete digestion of protein. You can be tested for polyamines through a simple urine test, the Indican test. It will confirm the need to lower your level of polyamines, which you can do through diet and taking proper supplements.

Also, with psoriasis and eczema, there is often an association with the presence of a bacterium called *Nanobacter*. This bacterium is about one thousand times smaller than regular bacteria and was only recently discovered by two researchers from Finland. (It is also commonly associated with coronary artery disease, kidney stones, polycystic kidney disease and prostate calcifications.) It is commonly present in individuals who have had root canals, periodontal disease or decayed, filled or missing teeth. It is also commonly found in vaccines.

> *And the LORD will remove from you all sickness; and He will not put on you any of the harmful diseases of Egypt which you have known, but He will lay them on all who hate you.*
> —DEUTERONOMY 7:15, NAS

If you follow the nutritional and dietary recommendations for psoriasis or eczema and still suffer from these disorders, I recommend that you be tested for Nanobacter. Medical Diagnostic Lab performs this test. You can call (856) 608-1696 to find a physician in your area to order the test. For more information on this topic, visit the website www.nanobaclabs.com.

Digestive enzymes and vitamin A

Two supplements especially helpful in decreasing polyamines are digestive enzymes and a vitamin A supplement. I recommend Divine Health Digestive Enzyme, which is an excellent product to aid digestion. Also, do not take more than 25,000 IU a day of vitamin A, and not more than 10,000 IU a day if you are pregnant. (Please see the back of this booklet for information on ordering Divine Health products.)

Gamma-linoleic acid (GLA)

Be sure to get enough gamma-linoleic acid. Taking evening primrose oil will supply your need for GLA. I recommend two tablets of Divine Health Evening Primrose Oil two times a day.

Fish oil (Omega-3 fatty acids)

Fish oil prevents the production of arachidonic acid, a major culprit in psoriasis and eczema. I recommend Divine Health Fish Oil, which contains 420 milligrams of EPA. Take two gel caplets two to three times per day. Supplementing Omega-3 fatty acids may be one of the most important things you can do for healing your skin. Divine Health Mega Omega contains a high dose of Omega-3 fatty acids and may result in a significant improvement in your skin disorder. Also, the fish oil is not rancid, as many that are in health food stores can be.

A comprehensive multivitamin

The rapid cell division in skin disorders can create nutritional deficiencies. In addition, patients with skin disorders usually have low levels of zinc and vitamin A, as well as deficiencies of B vitamins, selenium, chromium, vitamin E and other antioxidants. A comprehensive multivitamin will help to correct any vitamin and mineral deficiencies. I recommend a comprehensive multivitamin such as Divine Health Multivitamin.

L-glutamine

L-glutamine is an amino acid that improves intestinal permeability. It also feeds the cells of the small intestines. I recommend taking 500–1000 milligrams of L-glutamine thirty minutes before eating your meals. Another excellent supplement for repairing the GI tract is called Total Leaky Gut. It contains L-glutamine, N-acetyl glucosamine and DGL, as well as other nutrients that help to repair the GI tract. I recommend chewing one tablet of Total Leaky Gut thirty minutes before each meal for at least three months. This important supplement can be obtained by calling Nutri-West at (800) 451-5620.

Fiber

Another very important supplement for helping to prevent psoriasis is fiber, which helps to bind the toxins and excrete them in the feces, thus reducing the body's overall toxic burden.

The two main types of fiber are *soluble* and *insoluble*. Excessive amounts of soluble fiber, such as beans, psyllium seeds, peas and legumes, can actually lead to an overgrowth of intestinal bacteria, and thus may actually worsen psoriasis. *Insoluble fiber*, on the other hand, helps to inactivate many of the intestinal toxins. It also helps to prevent harmful bacteria and parasites from attaching themselves to the wall of your intestines by acting like a sweeping broom. An excellent insoluble fiber found in health food stores, microcrystalline cellulose, does not contain any wheat products and tends to be tolerated by those with sensitive GI tracts.

I usually recommend starting with 1 teaspoon

of fiber twice a day, usually mixed with water or a protein drink, and then gradually increasing up to 1 tablespoon twice a day.

Milk thistle

Milk thistle is a powerful herb that protects your liver from being damaged by toxic substances. It also helps restore glutathione levels, the most important antioxidant in the liver. I recommend 200 milligrams of milk thistle three times a day. Divine Health Milk Thistle is a pharmaceutical grade product that is extremely effective in detoxifying the liver.

Lecithin

Lecithin, which consists mainly of choline (a B vitamin), helps the body break down fat. It also helps the body absorb vitamin A through the intestines and even helps repair damage done to the liver by alcoholism. I mix granular lecithin with my protein drink twice a day. Granular lecithin can be found in any health food store and is inexpensive. Avoid lecithin if you are allergic to soy. I recommend 1 tablespoon of granular lecithin two or three times a day.

Herbal teas

Certain herbal teas, such as slippery elm bark

tea and saffron tea, are highly recommended for treating psoriasis. Dr. John O. A. Pagano, who has successfully treated many patients with severe cases of psoriasis, recommends drinking saffron tea before bedtime. Place ¼ teaspoon of saffron tea in a cup, and then pour boiling water over it. After letting it stand for fifteen to thirty minutes, strain it and drink it. I recommend adding a small amount of liquid Stevia to taste.

Dr. Pagano also recommends a cup of slippery elm bark tea in the early morning, approximately thirty minutes prior to breakfast. Make it fresh each time. He recommends placing ¼ teaspoon of slippery elm bark powder in a cup of warm water and letting it stand for about fifteen minutes prior to drinking it. Do not strain the slippery elm tea; it is a mucilage, which soothes inflamed mucous membranes of the bowels and is beneficial for most inflammatory conditions of the GI tract.

> *Yet it pleased the LORD to bruise him; he hath put him to grief: when thou shalt make his soul an offering for sin, he shall prolong his days.*
> —ISAIAH 53:10, KJV

Coenzyme Q-10

A comprehensive antioxidant formula containing both coenzyme Q-10 and lipoic acid are also important to help quench free radicals. Lipoic acid is the most important of all antioxidants since it recycles itself as well as coenzyme Q-10, vitamin C, vitamin E and glutathione. It also supports liver function, which is very important in patients with skin disorders.

Coenzyme Q-10 also has a prominent role in the production of energy in every cell of the body. Divine Health Advanced Antioxidant contains both lipoic acid and coenzyme Q-10 and should be taken once or twice a day in order to quench free radicals caused from toxic overload and compromised liver function.

Healing Supplements for Acne

A very inexpensive and effective treatment for acne is benzoyl peroxide, which can be purchased over the counter at your pharmacy. Benzoyl peroxide is an oxidizing agent that dries and peels the skin; it also helps to loosen impactions. For any acne treatment to be successful, the skin must become dry and peel. Expect it to become irritated. This means the medicine or treatment is penetrating into the pores and helping to break up and remove the impactions, releasing oxygen that kills the bacteria.

Benzoyl peroxide comes in three different strengths: 2.5 percent, 5 percent and 10 percent. For sensitive skin, start with the 2.5 percent strength once or twice a day. After a few weeks, you can increase the strength to the 5 percent. For normal skin, start with the 5 percent strength twice a day, and after a few weeks gradually increase it to 10 percent. (Note: Do not purchase benzoyl peroxide products that contain oil, since they are less effective.)

Rub benzoyl peroxide everywhere acne occurs, such as the nose, cheeks, chin, forehead and possibly the jaw line, as well as the back and chest. Avoid the area around the eyes, and also avoid the corner of the mouth and the area under the nostrils.

If your skin becomes too irritated, red and inflamed, simply lay off the benzoyl peroxide for a few days and give your skin a break. Don't start using moisturizers. Expect mild, but not severe, irritation.

I advise my patients to avoid oral antibiotics, which can cause candida overgrowth. Topically applied antibiotic lotions may be effective in some individuals, however.

Vitamin A

Vitamin A is a very healing supplement for acne as it normalizes the growth of skin cells and helps to remove impactions and prevent new ones from developing. However, vitamin A is potentially toxic at high doses, with serious side effects. Therefore, I do not recommend taking more than 25,000 IU per day or 10,000 IU daily for pregnant women.

I recommend a topical vitamin A prescription known as Retin-A. Besides providing the healing properties of vitamin A, the topical application will ensure that you avoid negative side effects caused by high doses of oral vitamin A. Use Retin-A only once a day, in the evening, after washing your face. Overuse can be very irritating to your skin.

> *Then Satan went out from the presence of the Lord, and smote Job with sore boils from the sole of his foot to the crown of his head.*
> —Job 2:7, NAS

If your skin gets red and irritated, stop the Retin-A for a few days and try using it every other day. Also, while using this product, avoid or dramatically limit sun exposure since Retin-A makes the skin more prone to sunburn. You can ask your family doctor or dermatologist to prescribe Retin-A. I prefer the Retin-A gel for my patients rather than the creams.

Zinc

A very important nutrient for treatment of acne is zinc. A zinc supplement may help decrease the inflammation in those with severe acne. I recommend zinc picolinate, approximately 50–100 milligrams a day.

Fiber

Taking a fiber supplement daily in the form of ground flaxseeds, psyllium or any other type of soluble fiber every day will be helpful, binding testosterone as well as other hormones in the GI tract and eliminating them from the body. That's important for acne because too much testosterone in the body, as is the case of many teens, triggers acne.

It's also important to take a fiber supplement daily to assure regular bowel movements each day. Many individuals with acne are constipated. Drinking two quarts of filtered water a day and taking a fiber supplement may dramatically improve acne conditions.

Azelaic acid

Azelaic acid is a natural product that is very effective for all forms of acne. It removes the impaction caused by the dead cells within the pore, and it has an antibacterial effect. Creams containing 20 percent azelaic acid have been shown to produce results equal to those of benzoyl peroxide, Retin-A and oral tetracycline.[2]

Azelaic acid should be applied to all acne-prone areas twice a day. I recommend choosing to use either benzoyl peroxide or

> *No evil will befall you, nor will any plague come near your tent.*
> —PSALM 91:10, NAS

azelaic acid, but not both. Expect to see results after using it for one month. You can ask your doctor to prescribe azelaic acid, or you may find it in some health food stores.

Alpha-hydroxy acids (AHA)

Alpha-hydroxy acids such as glycolic acid are fruit acids that can remove dead skin cells and stimulate the cells in the epidermis to produce new cells, which, interestingly, do not usually cause the impactions that lead to acne. Once the dead skin cells are removed with this product, the benzoyl peroxide, Retin-A or azelaic acid will actually work better.

A dermatologist or esthetician can administer a chemical peel containing these acids, or you can purchase alpha-hydroxy acids and glycolic acid at most cosmetic counters. Just make sure that that those cosmetic preparations do not contain any oils or other ingredients that can produce a breakout.

Selecting Your Personal Regimen

The following general classifications based on the severity of your acne condition will help you to choose your personal treatment regimen:

- Grade 1 acne—involves a few whiteheads and blackheads: Use only benzoyl peroxide or azelaic acid.

- Grade 2 acne—involves more whiteheads: Add Retin-A gel to the benzoyl peroxide or azelaic acid.

- Grade 3 acne—involves a mixture of blackheads, whiteheads and a number of inflammatory lesions; at least ten pimples or papules are constantly present: Add alpha-hydroxy acids to the benzoyl peroxide or azelaic acid and Retin-A gel.

- Grade 4 acne—involves cystic acne in addition to all of grade 3 eruptions: Use all the treatments included for Grade 3 acne, and see your dermatologist or family physician to add a *topical* antibiotic medication.

Stay on your acne regimen for two months *after* all of your lesions have cleared. Then begin a maintenance program by simply using either benzoyl peroxide or azelaic acid twice a day. If irritation occurs, decrease it to only once a day until you "outgrow" your tendency for acne.

If, after treating your acne condition faithfully with a combination of the above regimens, you do not see improvement, I recommend you get evaluated by a dermatologist to see if you are a candidate for Accutane, a powerful derivative of vitamin A. Use of this product must be closely monitored by your dermatologist.

Medical Therapies for Scarring

If your acne has left you with scars on your face, chest, back or shoulders, the following therapies may be helpful to alleviate the scarring effects:

- *Microdermabrasion* is performed by many estheticians or dermatologists to improve the appearance of wrinkles, acne scars and other unwanted marks.

- *Dermabrasion* is a more aggressive approach performed by certain dermatologists, and it involves use of a diamond disk rotating at high speeds to "sand" the tissues of the frozen epidermis. It gives wonderful results; you can usually expect a 50 to 80 percent improvement. There is some risk involved, so make sure you seek out an experienced dermatologist who has performed hundreds of these procedures.

Treatment for Acne Rosacea

If you have acne rosacea, you may need to increase the amount of hydrochloric acid in your stomach by taking betane HCL (150 milligrams) with each meal. Many individuals with rosacea do not produce adequate amounts of HCL.

Also, many patients with rosacea have both *helicobacter pylori* as well as GE reflux disease. Your primary care physician should examine you for both of these conditions. (For more information, refer to *The Bible Cure for Heartburn and Indigestion.*)

I recommend that you take a comprehensive multivitamin as well, like Divine Health Multivitamin. Metrogel is a topical antibiotic that is very effective for rosacea. However, it must be prescribed by your physician.

Following the same nutritional regimen as patients with psoriasis and eczema will bring positive results.

God Wants You Well

God wants you to feel well, look well and, most of all, to know His great love for you. Remember, the Bible says, "No one hates his own body but lovingly cares for it, just as Christ cares for his body, which is the church" (Eph. 5:29).

If you are a believer in Jesus Christ, you *are* the church. That means that He cherishes you with a greater love than your mind is able to fathom. Never let embarrassment or self-consciousness that can accompany a skin disorder cause you to forget that. You are loved!

A BIBLE CURE PRAYER
FOR YOU

Dear Lord, the apostle Paul prayed in Ephesians 3:18 to know how wide, how long, how high and how deep Your love is. Enlarge my capacity so that I will experience Your wonderful love and care for me. I believe that You cherish me, and I accept Your tender love. Thank You for Your gentleness toward me. I receive Your healing touch upon my body, even now. In Jesus' name, amen.

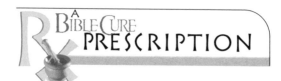

BIBLE CURE
PRESCRIPTION

Which category does your skin disorder fall into? How severe is it?

_____

_____

What supplements are you planning to begin taking to support your body in its healing process?

_____

_____

_____

_____

Look up Ephesians 3:18. Write it down in the space below and memorize it.

_____

_____

_____

Chapter 4

Lifestyle Choices

Your lifestyle choices can become a pathway of life and healing when you ask God for His help and direction. The psalmist declared, "Your word is a lamp for my feet and a light for my path" (Ps. 119:105). The Bible also promises, "He sent His word and healed them" (Ps. 107:20, NKJV). The words of wisdom in this booklet can be a healing message for you that God is sending your way. They can become light for your pathway as you choose to walk in the healing paths God has established for us. As you consider the lifestyle choices that follow, expect God to help you to choose the way that will bring you healing and health.

Healing Therapies for Psoriasis

A wonderful, and enjoyable, natural therapy for relieving psoriasis is exposure to sunlight, which has been used to treat psoriasis for hundreds of years. Sunlight can actually put your psoriasis into remission for weeks at a time.

A BIBLE CURE HEALTH TIP

Guidelines for Controlling Psoriasis With Sunlight

- Sunbathe before 11 A.M. and after 3 P.M., when the sun's rays are safer.

- Begin by sunbathing for five minutes on your back and another five minutes on your front, no more than ten minutes total time in the sun.

- Slowly increase your sun time to twenty to thirty minutes per side; just be sure that your skin is not burning.

If you have a fair complexion, use extra caution with sunlight because your skin will tend to be much more sensitive to the dangers of over-exposure. Too much sunlight can be extremely damaging to your skin, predisposing you to skin cancer. Ask your family doctor or dermatologist about a tanning program that's right for you.

Spending time in the sun has the added benefit of helping your body to make all the vitamin D it needs to help heal your skin. You may be not be aware that some people with severe psoriasis are very deficient in the active form of vitamin D. In 1993, a medication called Dovonex was released that provides a synthetic form of the natural vitamin D3. It is available to be applied twice a day as an ointment, cream or a solution for the scalp. You can ask your physician about it.

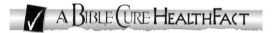

A BIBLE CURE HEALTHFACT

An Ancient Remedy

For hundreds of years, people who swam in the Dead Sea have received relief from psoriasis. The Dead Sea is thirteen hundred feet below sea level and contains a salt concentration ten times greater than the ocean. Trace elements of calcium, potassium, magnesium and bromine also aid healing. And the heavy atmosphere around the Dead Sea filters out harmful rays of the sun. Seventy to 80 percent of people who swim in the Dead Sea realize significant relief from their symptoms, some with remissions that last six months or longer.

HEALTHFACT HEALTHFACT HEALTHFACT HEALTHFACT HEALTHFACT HEALTHFACT HEALTHFACT

Medical treatments

Individuals with severe psoriasis are commonly given systemic medications including oral corticosteroids such as prednisone, methotrexate, cyclosporine and oral retinoids (for example, Soriatane and Accutane), which are derivatives of vitamin A. All of these medications are potentially very toxic and should be used only under the close supervision of your doctor. The natural therapies recommended in this book allow you to avoid the toxicities of systemic medications.

Healing Care for Acne-Prone Skin

Resisting the frustration involved with having less than "perfect" skin, you can learn to bring healing gently to your acne condition by becoming aware of the following healthy protocols.

Simple ways to avoid acne breakouts

- Avoid picking at your acne lesions since this aggravates more acne lesions and promotes scarring. When a pimple comes to a head with a white pustule, gently pressing the pustule to release the pore impaction will usually lead to clearing of the pimple. Ask your dermatologist or family doctor how to do this in a way that will avoid creating a scar.

- When your skin develops an inflamed papule, nodule or cyst that has not come to a head, avoid squeezing these lesions because that drives the inflammation deeper into the skin and results in a rupture of the follicular wall, creating even greater inflammation and scarring.

- Some people are prone to develop acne simply from resting their hand on their chin, cheek or forehead while studying, working at a computer or watching television.

- Wearing a headband, hat or a football helmet chinstrap can also promote acne.

- You can get acne behind the ears from wearing glasses.

- Acne can also erupt on the shoulders, back or chest from wearing a backpack or carrying a heavy purse on one shoulder. Frictional force, such as rubbing acne-prone skin, predisposes one to developing acne in those areas.

Cleansing acne-prone skin

A good acne treatment program starts with simply washing your face twice a day with an anti-bacterial soap and water. Be very careful to rinse your face thoroughly after washing. This will help to kill bacteria that are associated with acne.

However, don't get into the habit of scrubbing your face with a washcloth or using exfoliants that contain

> *He has caused my flesh and my skin to waste away.*
> —LAMENTATIONS 3:4, NAS

sandlike granules on the face, especially when pustules are present. Scrubbing and exfoliating cannot penetrate the impacted follicle and remove the impaction. Such rough treatment usually spreads acne instead of improving it.

Heat and humidity

Heat and high humidity may cause an acne outbreak. Humid summer weather, steam baths and saunas all may cause acne to flare up.

Occupational hazards for acne sufferers

Some occupations are worse for acne sufferers than others because they expose your skin to chemicals, cold tars and oils. Highway workers, roofers, refinery workers, auto mechanics and oil field workers are commonly exposed to petro-leum products, which can aggravate acne. Restaurant workers who must work around deep fryers and frying food are exposed to airborne grease and oils that can promote acne.

Anyone who must handle herbicides, insecti-cides and fungicides on the job can increase his or her risk of developing acne. I once had a patient who had acne cysts all over his chest and back and none on his face. His acne was caused by his job as a car detailer; he would lean against the cars while waxing them, and the car wax get-ting on his shirt would aggravate his acne.

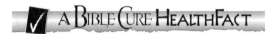

Medications That Promote Acne Breakouts

- Certain medications, such as corticos-teroids, are well-known culprits behind acne breakouts. These include prednisone as well as topical steroid creams, which may produce steroid acne.

- Acne is also common in men who take testosterone and anabolic steroids.

61

- Birth control pills that contain synthetic progesterones, levonorgestrel and norethisterone may cause acne to worsen. The newer progesterones, such as norgestimate, usually do not aggravate acne. Ortho Tri-cyclen is a birth control pill recommended for women with acne.

- Seizure medications such as Dilantin may also aggravate acne.

- Lithium, which is used for bipolar disorder, also aggravates acne.

- Illegal drugs can worsen acne, with one of the most common ones being marijuana.

Cautions with cosmetics

One of the most common aggravating factors for acne, especially in women, is cosmetics. Many popular skin care products and brands of makeup cause noninflammatory acne. You'll recall that this is the blackhead and whitehead type of acne that breaks out on the cheeks, chin and forehead.

Although it can take as long as six months to develop, when it happens, teenage girls can get into a vicious cycle by using more makeup in order to cover it up, which creates even more acne.

Making wise changes in your lifestyle according to the above information can help heal your acne prone skin dramatically.

Getting Relief for Eczema

A number of things you may be doing every day could be making your eczema much worse. For example, soaps, detergents and solvents can rob your skin of their natural oils, leaving them dry and easily damaged. Dry-cleaning fluids, paint thinners and other solvents and abrasive chemicals can worsen eczema.

To help combat this kind of damage, avoid regular soaps and use an olive oil cleanser, such as pure castile. You can find this in your local health food store. Be sure to apply moisturizers faithfully to your skin every day. The best time is right after your bath, since that's when the water content of your skin is highest.

A BIBLE CURE HEALTH TIP

Adding special oils to your bath water helps seal water into the skin. Sprinkle a few drops of some scented aromatherapy oil directly into your bath water. You can also apply olive oil directly to your skin after your bath. It's an excellent natural moisturizer.

If you suspect that your eczema is an allergic reaction, use mild detergent when washing clothes, and rinse the detergent thoroughly out of the clothes. Sometimes brands with borax are less irritating than stronger detergents. Also, use rubber gloves when washing dishes. Please refer to *The Bible Cure for Allergies* for more information concerning allergic reactions.

Fabrics and fibers

Wearing cotton fabric next to your skin and avoiding wool, nylon, polyester and other synthetic fabrics can relieve all forms of eczema.

If you have atopic dermatitis, you may find it helpful to place a cotton sheet over your fabric-covered couch or sofa. Leather rather than fabric furniture will be less irritating to your skin. If your child has eczema, cover the carpet with a cotton sheet before allowing your youngster to play on the floors where skin comes into contact with irritating carpet fibers.

Helpful humidity

Dry air and low humidity tend to make eczema worse. If you live in an area of the country where humidity tends to be very low, you will find that it helps your eczema to humidify your home. Heating your home during the winter months is also very drying; using a humidifier may provide welcome relief from eczema outbreaks.

As we have mentioned, drinking adequate amounts of water will keep the skin well hydrated, and using natural moisturizers will help keep the healing moisture in.

Stop scratching

Scratching away at itchy eczema will not bring the desired relief; it will usually make it worse. When necessary, take a natural antihistamine such as quercetin (500 milligrams three times a day) or an over-the-counter antihistamine such as Benadryl. Your family doctor may also prescribe an appropriate antihistamine to help relieve the itching. Zinc oxide applied to the skin also helps to control itching.

Many children with eczema develop recurrent skin infections, usually from scratching. Good skin care, as well as controlling scratching and itching, goes a long way in helping to prevent secondary skin infections. In children, as well as adults, keeping fingernails short will minimize the damage caused by scratching, especially during the night while sleeping.

Following a Wise Pathway to Health

I encourage you to commit the way you think and the lifestyle choices you make involving your skin care to God. He cares about everything in your life, even your skin. He will help you to choose a wise pathway toward a healthy lifestyle.

The Bible says that He cares so much about you that you could not even count the number of thoughts He has had about you today (Ps. 139:17). So, accept His wise counsel and loving guidance for all of your daily lifestyle choices, and you will enjoy the health He promises to give.

A BIBLE CURE PRAYER
FOR YOU

Dear Lord, I boldly choose to trust in You and Your loving provision for all my needs—especially for the health of my skin. I trust in You and ask You to direct my path by leading me in a godly course of action for my skin disorder. I commit my way to You as the scripture says in Proverbs 3:5, and I ask for You to guide my path. In Jesus' name, amen.

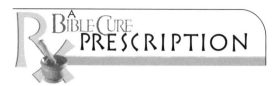

BIBLE CURE PRESCRIPTION

How do you think about your skin? Do you have kind, caring thoughts about it, or are they harsh and resentful?

_____

_____

Write a prayer asking God's forgiveness for not loving and appreciating the skin He's given to you. Ask Him for more godly attitudes about your skin.

_____

_____

_____

Now, write a prayer thanking God for helping you to overcome your skin disorder, even before it's completely healed.

_____

_____

_____

Chapter 5

Triumphing Through Faith

Faith works like a powerful shield to protect you from the forces all around you that might tear down your health and strength—body, soul and spirit. In Jesus Christ you can live shielded in the impenetrable might of bold, living faith. The Bible says, "In every battle you will need faith as your shield to stop the fiery arrows aimed at you by Satan" (Eph. 6:16). Again, in Proverbs 30:5 we read, "He is a shield unto them that put their trust in him" (KJV).

Even if you've never considered doing so, I encourage you to begin to apply faith to your situation. Declaring the Word of God in faith becomes an awesome force against every disease and affliction—body, soul and spirit.

Is Your Skin Weeping?

I'll never forget the words of a psychiatry professor I had in medical school. He had previously been a dermatologist for years and had treated numerous psoriasis sufferers. On one occasion I approached him and asked why he left the field of dermatology to study psychiatry. His answer overwhelmed me then, and it still does to this day. He said that his work as a dermatologist led him to conclude that many individuals suffering with skin disorders were actually "weeping through their skin." He wanted to study to get to the root of their problem.

Focus on the Roots

Although we have discussed the natural causes of skin disorders, it is also possible that a deeper root of your problem involves emotional pain. Perhaps you should ask the Holy Spirit to show you a psychological root cause of your skin disorder. Ask yourself:

- Am I overly stressed?

- Have I been really frustrated lately?

- Am I angry with a person? At life?

- Am I feeling overwhelmed?

Emotional pain is a powerful force, and it can be a root of many skin disorders—even those that seem to be simply physical in nature. To experience complete and long-term healing, it's vital that you investigate the possibility that the cause of your skin disorder may have spiritual roots. However, do so in faith and with great hope, because the Word of God promises to heal our emotional and spiritual pain (Luke 4:18).

The Bible says, "Every plant not planted by my heavenly Father will be rooted up" (Matt. 15:13). I believe that any deep,

> *Ye know how through infirmity of the flesh I preached the gospel unto you.*
> —GALATIANS 4:13, KJV

hidden roots of emotional pain will be yanked up by the loving, healing work of the precious Holy Spirit. So today I join my faith with yours, believing for a powerful work of the Holy Spirit in your life.

The Stigma of Leprosy

Some people consider skin disorders to be a modern kind of leprosy that proves God is against them and is judging them as He did Miriam when she criticized her brother Moses. (See Numbers 12.) They forget that God also healed Miriam of her leprosy in answer to Moses' prayer. God is a merciful, loving God who has made provision for our health, but sometimes we need to forgive someone in our past who has hurt us.

You must come to know that God loves you and deeply desires that your life might be free from all pain and every affliction. Begin to expect a miracle; expect God to heal you!

Building Faith for a Miracle

The Bible says, "Faith comes from listening to this message of good news—the Good News about Christ" (Rom. 10:17). Reading the Bible and choosing to believe God's powerful Word will create faith in your heart.

Know that the Bible is not just a book of words; it's a book of God's mighty words. As such, it has power to transform your spirit and redeem your soul and body. As you read, the Word of God can transform your thinking so that you are released from angry, frustrated and painful thoughts (Rom. 12:2). You can begin thinking true thoughts of God's love for you and find rest for your souls (Matt. 11:28). And you can begin to confess the reality of your healing (1 Pet. 2:24).

As you dwell on the goodness of God, your attitude toward your skin disorder will change from hopelessness and frustration to hope and faith that allow you to imagine your skin totally healed and whole—clean and clear as a baby's flesh.

Declare by faith: *I believe that my skin is totally healed of all symptoms of my skin disorder.* Then dare to declare Jesus' words: "You can pray for anything, and if you believe, you will have it" (Mark 11:24).

You Have to Tell Somebody

As your skin begins to clear, be sure to tell someone. As you share your testimony of the healing power of God you are experiencing, not only will it help them, but it will strengthen your faith as well. And the Bible says we overcome through the blood of the lamb and the power of our testimony (Rev. 12:11).

Give Thanks

Gratitude is a powerful, healing attitude that reinforces the blessing of our healing. When God heals you, it is important to bow your heart and tell God that you are truly and genuinely grateful. The Bible teaches us to give thanks!

Learn to Love and Accept Your Skin

Learn to love and accept your skin as your best friend. Learn to appreciate it as the protective covering that God has given you. I have had diabetic patients who had numbness in their feet. Because of the numbness, they didn't experience pain when they should have, and as a result, some even had to have their toes or feet amputated due to infection. The ultimate cause was the malfunction of their skin.

Listen to your skin; don't ignore it. Be kind to it by helping it to heal. The Bible says to love one another as

Even when I remember, I am disturbed, and horror takes hold of my flesh.
—Job 21:6, NAS

you love yourself. (See Matthew 19:19.) Loving your skin is one aspect of loving yourself. Too many of us curse our skin and our bodies through our words and attitudes.

God made us to be temples of the Holy Spirit (1 Cor. 3:16–17). That means His blessing rests within our physical bodies. As we honor Him, we will learn to honor our bodies and treat them lovingly.

When you love your body, you will begin

giving it the foods and nutritional supplements it needs. It will be a genuine pleasure to choose the pathway of healing for your skin disorder. That is the attitude the Holy Spirit will give you toward your body, and you will stop making your skin disorder worse with poor nutrition. Love is the most powerful healing force in the universe, so begin applying it. Start loving yourself as you love others!

Conclusion

As a doctor, I've seen far more pain and suffering than most people have. I've also been privileged to witness God's healing power at work in the lives of His precious people as well. Those individuals who simply believe in God's mercy and trust in His wonderful love are never disappointed. If you will only step out in faith, you too will witness the power of God in your own life. Just remember, He loves you more than you could ever know. So, choose faith. You'll be glad you did!

A BIBLE CURE PRAYER
FOR YOU

Dear Lord, teach me how to walk in powerful, living faith—the faith that overcomes every obstacle. I'm beginning today in a new walk of faith by proclaiming my healing: I thank You, Lord Jesus, that by Your stripes I'm healed of my skin disorder.

I thank You for delivering me of even the roots of spiritual pain and hidden emotion. You are so good and such a wonderful, loving Father. I give You thanks for all You've done in my life. And Lord, I promise to begin loving myself and treating my skin with the tender love that You intended. In Jesus' name, amen.

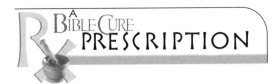

Write how you see your skin through the eyes of faith.

_____

_____

Go through this Bible Cure booklet and find seven Scripture verses that really speak to you about your condition. Write the references out below.

_____

_____

_____

_____

Write your own prayer of thanksgiving, thanking God for loving and healing you.

_____

_____

_____

A PERSONAL NOTE

From Don and Mary Colbert

God desires to heal you of disease. His Word is full of promises that confirm His love for you and His desire to give you His abundant life. His desire includes more than physical health for you; He wants to make you whole in your mind and spirit as well through a personal relationship with His Son, Jesus Christ.

If you haven't met my best friend, Jesus, I would like to take this opportunity to introduce Him to you. It is very simple.

If you are ready to let Him come into your heart and become your best friend, just bow your head and sincerely pray this prayer from your heart:

Lord Jesus, I want to know You as my Savior and Lord. I believe You are the Son of God and that You died for my sins. I also believe You were raised from the dead and now sit at the right hand of the Father praying for me. I ask You to forgive me for my sins and change my heart so that I can

be Your child and live with You eternally.
Thank You for Your peace. Help me to
walk with You so that I can begin to know
You as my best friend and my Lord. Amen.

If you have prayed this prayer, we rejoice with you in your decision and your new relationship with Jesus. Please contact us at pray4me@strang.com so that we can send you some materials that will help you become established in your relationship with the Lord. You have just made the most important decision of your life. We look forward to hearing from you.

Notes

PREFACE:

THERE'S A CLEANSING FOUNTAIN

1. Acne Information Package, National Institute of Arthritis and Musculoskeletal and Skin Diseases, DHEW Publication No. (HRA) 76-1639.

CHAPTER 1:

CLOTHED WITH WISDOM

1. Joseph Pizzorno and Michael Murray, *Textbook of Natural Medicine,* Vol. 2 (New York: Churchill Livingstone, 1999).

2. Clayton L. Thomas, M.D., M.P.H., editor, *Taber's Cyclopedic Medical Dictionary* (Philadelphia: F. A. Davis Company, 1997), s.v. "acne."

3. Anthony Chu, *The Good Skin Doctor* (Hammersmith, London: Thorsens, 1999).

CHAPTER 2:

GLOWING THROUGH NUTRITION

1. A. W. Burks et al., "Peanut Protein as a Major Cause of Adverse Food Reaction in Patients with Atopic Dermatitis," *Allergy Proceedings* 10 (1989): 265–269.

CHAPTER 3:

BEAUTIFYING WITH SUPPLEMENTS

1. John O. A. Pagano. *Healing Psoriasis* (Englewood Cliffs, NJ: The Pagano Organization, Inc, 2000).

2. M. Nazzaro-Porro, "Azelaic Acid," *Jam Acad Dermatol* 17 (1987): 1033–1041.

BIBLE CURE

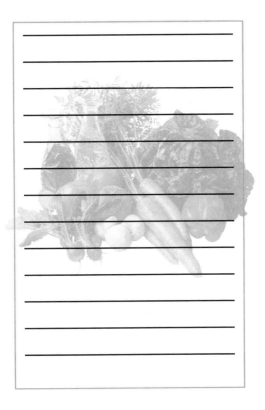

_____
_____
_____
_____
_____
_____
_____
_____
_____
_____
_____
_____
_____

BIBLE CURE

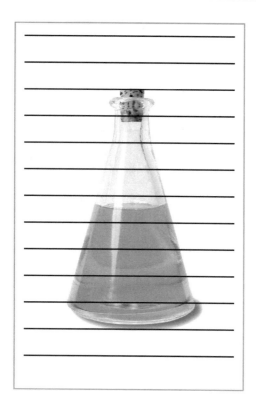

_____
_____
_____
_____
_____
_____
_____
_____
_____
_____
_____
_____

BIBLE CURE

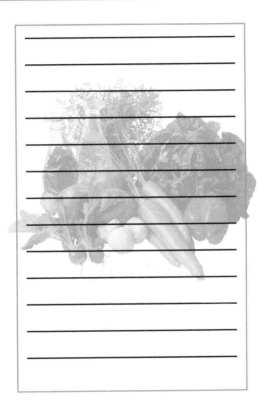

_____
_____
_____
_____
_____
_____
_____
_____
_____
_____
_____
_____

BIBLE CURE

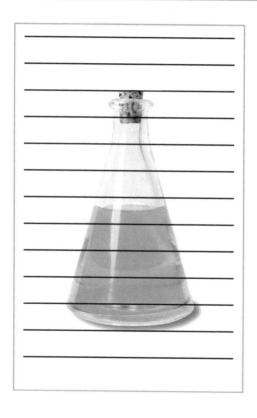

NOTES

_____

_____

_____

_____

_____

_____

_____

_____

_____

_____

_____

_____

_____

Don Colbert, M.D., was born in Tupelo, Mississippi. He attended Oral Roberts School of Medicine in Tulsa, Oklahoma, where he received a bachelor of science degree in biology in addition to his degree in medicine. Dr. Colbert completed his internship and residency with Florida Hospital in Orlando, Florida. He is board certified in family practice and has received extensive training in nutritional medicine.

If you would like more
information about natural and
divine healing, or information about
Divine Health Nutritional Products ®,
you may contact
Dr. Colbert at:

DR. DON COLBERT

1908 Boothe Circle
Longwood, FL 32750
Telephone: 407-331-7007
(For ordering products only)

Dr. Colbert's website is
www.drcolbert.com.

Disclaimer: Dr. Colbert and the staff of Divine Health Wellness Center are prohibited from addressing a patient's medical condition by phone, facsimile or e-mail. Please refer questions related to your medical condition to your own primary care physician.

Pick up these other Siloam Press
books by Dr. Colbert:

Toxic Relief

Walking in Divine Health

What You Don't Know May Be Killing You

The Bible Cure® Booklet Series

The Bible Cure for ADD and Hyperactivity
The Bible Cure for Allergies
The Bible Cure for Arthritis
The Bible Cure for Back Pain
The Bible Cure for Cancer
The Bible Cure for Candida and Yeast Infection
The Bible Cure for Chronic Fatigue and Fibromyalgia
The Bible Cure for Depression and Anxiety
The Bible Cure for Diabetes
The Bible Cure for Headaches
The Bible Cure for Heart Disease
The Bible Cure for Heartburn and Indigestion
The Bible Cure for Hepatitis and Hepatitis C
The Bible Cure for High Blood Pressure
The Bible Cure for Irritable Bowel Syndrome
The Bible Cure for Memory Loss
The Bible Cure for Menopause
The Bible Cure for Osteoporosis
The Bible Cure for PMS and Mood Swings
The Bible Cure for Prostate Disorders
The Bible Cure for Skin Disorders
The Bible Cure for Sleep Disorders
The Bible Cure for Stress
The Bible Cure for Weight Loss and Muscle Gain

SILOAM PRESS

A part of Strang Communications Company
600 Rinehart Road
Lake Mary, FL 32746
(800) 599-5750